THE DOCTOR'S PRESCRIPTION FOR WHAT'S AILING AMERICA

VANCE ALM, MD

outskirts
press

The Doctor's Prescription for What's Ailing America
All Rights Reserved.
Copyright © 2019 Vance Alm, MD
v2.0

The opinions expressed in this manuscript are solely the opinions of the author and do not represent the opinions or thoughts of the publisher. The author has represented and warranted full ownership and/or legal right to publish all the materials in this book.

This book may not be reproduced, transmitted, or stored in whole or in part by any means, including graphic, electronic, or mechanical without the express written consent of the publisher except in the case of brief quotations embodied in critical articles and reviews.

Outskirts Press, Inc.
http://www.outskirtspress.com

ISBN: 978-1-9772-0069-3

Cover Photo © 2019 Vance Alm, MD. All rights reserved - used with permission.

Outskirts Press and the "OP" logo are trademarks belonging to Outskirts Press, Inc.

PRINTED IN THE UNITED STATES OF AMERICA

Table of Contents

Preface

This book is intended to start a conversation about a plan that would change health care in this country. It is not intended to be the definitive answer to all questions regarding such a system, and it will not have every statistical number or definition of ideas that will be discussed. This is my presentation of an alternative health care system. Additional facts, figures, and examples from life may be included in a future edition, but this short book is intended to get the idea out, so discussion may begin. I invite you to utilize this book as a foundation upon which you can begin your own conversations of where you think we, as a nation, should be headed to fix the critical problems related to health care in America.

Introduction

"Yes, health care in America is broken!" That was the answer from 100% of the people that I asked the simple question, "Is health care broken, and are there areas that need to be fixed?" I stopped asking after getting hundreds of answers to the affirmative. I recently traveled to Europe and asked a similar question, "What do you think of your country's health care system?" I expected that the responses would be a rather bland, "Oh, it's okay." In the UK I got these unexpected answers: "It's awesome, I don't know what I would have done during my cancer scare." "It's excellent but I'm worried, there is talk of privatization." And from a 28-year old guy in London, "It's f…ing great, man!" Those were not the answers I had expected, because there are so many articles describing how awful and inefficient the UK system is, and that the care is substandard and requires excessive wait times. I then traveled to France and met a man who had emigrated from the UK. I figured he would probably think that the UK system must be better than where he was. Again, I was surprised when he said that, though the UK system was good, the French medical system was superior to the UK system. When in Norway, I asked a server what she felt about Norway's system? "It's much better than my native country of Sweden. It's probably the best in Europe." Every person that I talked to in Europe, no matter which country, insisted that their country's health system was superior to the other countries.

How is it that the Europeans all appreciate and enjoy their system and yet? In the US, every person says that our health care system is broken and needs to be fixed! The simple answer is that Europe has embraced the fact that their government can provide care for the people of their country more effectively, more efficiently, and at a lower cost than we do in the US. These countries provide health care at little or no additional cost to their citizens. Many people would declare, "Free health care, why that's preposterous, it simply can't be done! Who would pay for it?" How much is spent on health care in countries around the world? The US spends, on average, about $9,000 per person, per year. That's the average for all health care for every person in the US. The average for most developed countries is about a third of that, only $3,000 per person. Most of that cost is paid by the government through taxes, not the individual's own pocketbook.

While many in the US are emphatic that they wouldn't stand to be taxed for their health care, in fact, we already do pay for government health care plans. Medicare and Medicaid cost the federal government about $1 trillion per year. Add in Public Health Service, Indian Health Service, the VA, and Military Medicine and it's even more! Much, if not most, of that money is going through commercial health care facilities, which tend to be less efficient, have much higher costs and focus on profit rather than health. That's why total costs for health care in the US are roughly $3.3 trillion, when you've added in the $2.3 trillion of personal and business payments for insurance premiums, copays, deductibles. Yet, if we were to set up a system like the UK has, with government owning and running all the operations, we would likely spend closer to $3,000 per person. If that were done, then we could have the system for less than what the nation spends for just Medicare and Medicaid. ($3,000 per person times 330 million Americans is $990 billion — that's less than the $1 trillion currently being spent!) If we just examine costs of the US medical system, then it is time to further evaluate a true public health care system and save money on the nation's better health!

Many people assume that because we spend so much money on health care, people living in the US must have the best health. Many believe that government run health systems just couldn't provide for good health. Sadly, if we look to two key indicators of a nation's health, life expectancy and infant mortality, then the US is not getting its money's worth, in relation to our nation's health. Life expectancy at birth is one statistic; we rank 43 out of over 200 nations in the world. I personally don't think that's very respectable for the greatest nation on earth. We're not first? We're not even in the top 40! How can that be? We live to a fairly respectable age of 79.5, but that is about 5 years less than the people of Hong Kong who live to 84.46 years. What's even worse is that our life expectancy has declined over the last two years. So, we may not live as long, but we probably do great at the beginning of life, right? Looking at infant mortality, the rate of infants born in the US who die before age one, paints an even grimmer picture. The highest death rates are in Africa, the lowest rates are in east Asia (Japan, Singapore, Hong Kong, and South Korea). The US comes in at number 55 of 225. At least we're ahead of Russia by 8 spots. These two statistics underscore the fact that we are not getting our money's worth! Health care in America is broken. The countries that lead us in these statistics all have one thing in common: a national health care system of some type. It seems from just the few facts so far, that a national health plan does have merit. That it could be cheaper and provide better results are very compelling reasons to consider this as an option.

Have I piqued your interest in this other option for health care? Let's look at what else might persuade you to consider this new national public health care system. If it cost most Americans less, would that be a compelling reason to consider a change to our current system? We currently have a system that has insurance companies reimbursing providers and facilities for our health care bills. The federal government is one of the larger "insurance providers" with Medicare and Medicaid, but individuals and corporations pay dearly for commercial insurance plans. We, the people paying for commercial health insurance, are each responsible for paying about $6,000 per year for our portion of our insurance coverage costs. Corporations (employers) are on the hook for about $12,000 per employee, per year. Then there are deductibles: $500, $1,000, $5,000, even $12,000. You must pay that amount before you even start getting your insurance coverage! Oh, and don't forget your co-pays, out of network costs, non-covered benefits; those really add up. The US is the only country that penalizes people for becoming sick and then forces them into bankruptcy to cover their health care costs. It's time to get away from the commercial insurance system and have quality health care provided directly by the federal government.

So far, my discussion has primarily centered on cost. "Who's going to pay for health care?" Politicians argue back and forth as to whether the government should be responsible to pay for health care. Personally, I believe that health care should be a right of every person in this country, and that it is the responsibility of the government to care for each of us. The Affordable Care Act was intended to guarantee access to health care. It improved access, but it was imperfect. More important is the fact that it failed to address all the other problems in health care. Cost seemed to be just the tip of the iceberg as far as problems with health care. The responses by politicians seem to be short sighted and strictly partisan. Costs are important, but who can determine the value of one person's life? We fail to recognize that other problems are continuing to drive those costs even higher. The belief is that health care costs simply rise to the level that the market will bear. This would be assuming that the health care system is a free market; it is not! When you or your loved one are suffering from chest pains, you are not going to shop around for the best bargain. Few people are going to question that, if they are to live, they must pay the hospital's price. It is extremely difficult to determine the value of one person's life. Life is not something most of us will bargain for. We generally are quite agreeable to pay whatever the cost is to stay alive. The current system has few cost comparisons or even tables of what the costs might be. Even with that, there are few people who would be willing to go to the cheapest hospital for fear they would not receive the "Best" care possible. You are much more likely to go to the closest care facility, no matter the cost. Because of that willingness to pay, profit motive will continue to drive costs up. Current projections are that the increase will continue at roughly 5% per year. Multiply that times the current estimate for health care costs, $3.3 trillion, and you have an increase of $165 billion every year. Those amounts are staggering, and our nation cannot bear them much longer. The medical share of the GDP is 18%, which means one out of every six dollars spent in this country is now for health care. If nothing is done, then health care will soon be the only product we produce. It's time to make a change, before health care bankrupts our country.

As you can see, I strongly believe that we must make fundamental changes to the US health care system. Health care is a major concern for everyone at some time in their life, and I believe that it can be provided better, more efficiently, and at less cost than our current for-profit system. In this book I will present the who, what, where, how, and why of the change I envision. Just like a good reporter, I hope to present the information that will persuade you to see the merits of a government provided health care system.

As I mentioned previously, cost is a major reason to change to such a system, however, there are many other reasons as well. When this new system is implemented there will be a transition period while changes are implemented. When the components are in place, I believe that most people and businesses will switch to this new federal health care system. Most likely, a hybrid system, using both private and government care, would continue after implementing this new system. There would be a national system providing most of the health care in the country, and a commercial system would also continue for those willing to pay the higher costs of a private system. The federal medical care plan would be the public option for care in this country; guaranteed at no additional cost to the patient. Those who do not partake in this system would not receive tax breaks for not utilizing it. The options would be: no-additional cost for federal health care, or the use of commercial health care, with no penalties for the use of either system.

The proposal I am suggesting consists of my initial concept for a different way of accessing health care. This concept is intended to be an overview of what a federal medical system might look like. I hope this idea will inspire true discussion about the problems in health care and how they might best be overcome. In the following chapters, you will be presented with a new national health care system — a Federal Medicine system. Or, as I prefer to call it, Fed Med.

The Concept

THE BASICS OF this new health care system, Fed Med, would be this: The US would purchase and maintain federal health care facilities and hire government health care providers (salaried government doctors) to provide health care directly to you. Fed Med is health care provided directly to every person in this country. There would be decreased administrative costs as you omit the added expense and necessity of insurance. This would eliminate the middleman from interfering with, or hindering, your access to care. If you are ill or are injured, you simply go to the federal medical facility and get treated. Our doctors would be hired by the people (through the federal government) to provide care directly to the people of our country. Of the people, for the people!

Most of the developed world already practices some form of government supplied health care, as they have recognized the responsibility of a government to provide for a healthy populace. Thus, people and the nation are healthier and stronger. A government supplied program is direct health care without layers of administrative bureaucracy blocking access to care. This program provides access to affordable, high quality health care for everyone who wants to use this system. There would be no mandatory use, just an offer for high quality care without additional cost. Just as we expect the government to protect us from external threats through a strong military, we should expect the government to provide for the health and well being of its citizens with an excellent health care system. Health care should be a right of the people from a government performing its duty to care for its citizens. Fed Med is the best choice for your future health care.

Health care provided by the government sounds great. But let's get back to the primary concern of many politicians, "How are you going to pay for it?" — "How much is it going to cost?" The government is going to provide this great service to you, but will they have to require payment for the service provided? The concept of no additional cost for health care seems impossible to attain. The nation is currently spending $1.1 trillion on Medicare and Medicaid. By applying those funds instead, directly to the new program, the US will be able to cover the costs with no additional cost to you, the patient. That sum, $1.1 trillion dollars, is over 60% of the national budget. The federal government is spending more than one million-millions (that's what $1 trillion is!) on health care, and that is just the Medicare and Medicaid portion. That money is spent mostly on the commercial (for profit) side of medicine: the hospitals, clinics, and doctors. We, as taxpayers are paying for a system that makes huge profits for insurance companies and big health systems while not providing a quality product. That is the problem with our current system, and why there would be so much resistance to change. Too many people are making lots of money to provide your health care and they aren't giving us very good results. Health care, right now, is big — BIG business. In the past in the US, and in other countries now, the emphasis was on keeping people as healthy as possible, decreasing suffering, and to treating disease. It seems that the emphasis now is how the health care and insurance industry will generate more money, more profit, and more income to the hospitals, insurance and providers. When those groups talk about lowering costs, it is often not to reduce patient cost but it really represents the means to reduce costs and expenditures, so the resulting efficiencies will result in greater profit for the health industry.

Our nation's health care mission statement must revolve around and emphasize the health of each of you, our citizens. Unfortunately, the mission statements of too many current business entities is, "Providing the best possible care while controlling costs". Let's get rid of the second half of those mission statements and simply focus on "Providing the best care that results in the optimum health of our patients." You deserve the emphasis to be on health, and you deserve to know that everything possible is being done to enhance the outcome of your health. You deserve to know that the part of the mission statement that says, "controlling costs", is for your benefit, as opposed to the bottom line of the corporation. If cost control is important, then it should be for the benefit of you, the patient, to reduce your costs for care or your insurance costs. Too often the control of costs is to benefit the corporation; so that they will be able to enhance their profits, earnings per share or management bonuses. The evidence points to making more money, with less concern about the welfare of the patients. That profit motive is what has turned medicine into an industry rather than the art of caring for you, the citizens of this great country. The way the current system is set up, it is increasingly difficult for many of us, as physicians, to stay true to compassion and caring. We are too often compelled to become part of corporate medicine; and then start seeing more patients in less time, doing more procedures, and billing at the highest code level we can. It's time to take the profit motive out of medicine and return to a focus on your health.

One of the biggest profit generators is the insurance industry. Insurance was originally brought forth to provide a benefit to workers to entice them to a work place when wage increases were banned in World War II industries. The concept that an employee would not have to pay to see the doctor was a new perk. Now, sadly insurance has become indispensable with the huge costs of health care. It is no longer just a welcome perk but is now a necessary requirement for living in the US. It has helped to drive costs higher as we felt it wasn't necessary to monitor health care costs because insurance was supposed to help us take care of those costs. Insurance is now a mandatory cost, that everyone is required to have, even though insurance companies do not provide health care. That cost, of insurance coverage, is now one of the driving factors in the debates regarding health care. The politicians go around and around debating how and who is going to pay for health care, and in end the government payments from your taxes usually get funneled through the for-profit systems. If we were to just have the federal government take over care, then the question is answered, and there is no need for insurance. If the government owned the facilities, and the providers were employees of the government, then payment is already done. The patient, that is you, would no longer need worry about ability to pay, and the provider doesn't worry about how she will get paid. The patient checks in, is triaged and care is provided. You as a patient can get the care you need when you need it. I mentioned triaging, this is assigning the case to the appropriate level of care; emergent, urgent or routine. Emergent is that life or loss of limb type of problem that must be treated immediately, such as a heart attack or accident that has damaged you. Urgent is pressing problems that will worsen if not treated soon or need to address control of pain, such as a bronchitis progressing to pneumonia or new onset knee pain after playing football at school. Then routine care requiring follow up to ensure that the problem remains controlled or treated, such as high blood pressure or depression. We currently have a system that pushes patients to use emergency care, because it pays the hospital more. We have a system that ensures that no one can be turned away from emergency care, so that there is always a provider of last resort, but again this inflates the cost of care. If we had a government system, we could reduce this expensive aspect of care by using appropriate levels of care. We would speed up access, because there would be less need for administrative check in and researching eligibility to receive care. If you are human and are in the US, then your eligibility is already taken as fact and you get your care. Everyone in the country is eligible. Unfortunately for too many people, that step of checking eligibility results in huge out of pocket expenses. Often even when you have "good" insurance you still end up with copays, the deductible and other costs. This worry over these additional costs often causes people to delay seeking medical care until it is a severe problem. Many people instead of seeking care when the problem is minor, will often wait until it is severe and often much costlier and more difficult to treat. Insurance is not the same for everyone. There are so many different companies, all with different rules from one another and often having different rules for different plans, depending on their cost. Medicaid and Medicare, the government's current insurance plans, each have another set of completely different rules and regulations. The difference is most often noticed in which providers are available for you to utilize, which treatments are considered covered benefits and which medicines are on your formulary, the insurance company's list of medicines. These differences result in greatly different treatment in the current medical system. The result is that often insurance ends up being just a piece of paper with a promise to pay for care, often it works well but too frequently it has financially catastrophic results. You, the patient, can often have a very different expectation or understanding of what the insurance company will pay. In some situations that paper promise ends up being worthless, because a patient would be unable to travel to the covered provider or the insurance dictates only certain providers that have long wait times. The promise of treatment disappears. Another complaint about insurance is the far too common phrase, "but I thought I was covered!" You, the patient are then forced to pay most or all of the cost of their care, as if you didn't even have health insurance.

Fed Med, or government provided care, could provide real, quality health care to everyone in this country. It would be able to provide care for less than what we pay for Medicaid and Medicare because there is no need of generating a profit. Its entire reason for existence is just to provide quality care to enhance the health of everyone in this country. Insurance would likely become a thing of the past, as more and more people shift to a public health care system like I envision. Those awful limits placed on health care by insurance would also disappear. We would get actual care from our government, not just a paper promise for care. We can do better with our health care and government supplied care is the best way to improve the health and wellbeing for the people of this country.

To summarize, here are some of the concepts currently being discussed:

1. The Affordable Care Act (Obama Care)

   - many providers don't take the insurance provided by the act or Medicaid

   - insurance premiums have risen far faster than the forecast rates.

- there are still too many people that still are not insured

- it does nothing to address many of the problems that are present in our current medical system

2. Repeal the Affordable Care Act

   - this option leaves between 11 and 13 million Americans without coverage

3. Warren Buffet, Jeff Bezos and a Wall Street banker plan

   - to build their own health care corporation to supply their employees with care directly from their corporation because current system costs are too high

4. Medicare for All

   - plan to provide care by giving Medicare coverage to everyone

   - it continues to use the current system, which is inefficient and is still driven by profit motive

   - there remain no means to control cost increases

   - it would bankrupt the country, if estimates of current Medicare costs are applied and then extrapolated to cover the entire US population

- it does nothing to address the other problems in our current medical system such as putting more facilities in rural areas

5. Do nothing, assume everything is OK

   - the country will go bankrupt as the cost of health care consumes more and more of the government, business and personal budgets

   - the lack of providers, rural facilities and mental health care remain unaddressed

6. Medical Care for a Healthy Society (or as I call it, Fed Med)

   - no additional cost to the patient/consumer, the new system would be paid for using funds that are currently spent by the government through Medicaid and Medicare

   - no more insurance premiums for individuals or corporations

   - a tremendous boost to the economy as those funds are now available for other expenditures

   - no qualifying for coverage, direct care for everyone is covered through government facilities

- this system would address many of the other problems facing healthcare

- increased mental health care

- improved access through the following:

    - more rural and inner-city facilities

    - more providers

    - specialists based on need, not profit

- this plan would better address the opioid crisis

- it would cost less! $0.8-1.5 trillion versus $3.1 trillion that the country spends now

The Facilities for Fed Med

PEOPLE WILL ASK, "Where would a federal medical system be located?" Currently there are over 4000 commercial, private and public hospitals in the US. That number fluctuates somewhat as some facilities are opening while others close. Consolidations, mergers, newer facilities, closing facilities due to age of the structure and closings due to non-profitability or not enough people using the facility, those are some of the reasons for closures. There are often multiple brands (competing facilities) within a geographic region and commonly no facilities in small towns as they were deemed inefficient or providers would not locate to those small towns. The federal government has already helped to establish different tiers of care, according to the level of care that can be provided at a facility, especially regarding trauma and burn care. Fed Med would likely have a similar hierarchy of care, but there would be an emphasis on placing at least some form of care closer to the patients, particularly rural or remote areas. This is similar to the manner in which military medicine is practiced, in that a medic or corpsman is placed in each company, so that basic care is available at the lowest level. Then each level will have increasing capabilities, so they can care for a wider range of problems. As a patient problem became more complicated or difficult to manage it could be moved to the next level of care. This is similar to current commercial medicine, but placement of facilities is often based on profitability not proximity to patient need. Progress in care often starts with the primary care provider and then transferred to a specialist's office, then to the hospital and possibly to a specialty hospital if the complexity warrants these transfers for patient need. In our current system a side entryway to this pattern is through the Emergency Room. This is often the place for all levels of care, resulting in packed waiting rooms, as everyone is required to be seen in Emergency Rooms. A government facility could triage care better and put patients in the level of care they truly need, if an emergent, life threatening problem then they would be treated immediately. If urgent, the care could be shifted to a different care provider, leaving the emergency provider free to handle truly emergency cases (those that are life threatening or have a threat of loss of limb). Protocols for rapid movement of a patient, requiring increased level of care, would quickly move a patient to level of care needed for the presenting problems. This triaging would allow for a more efficient and effective treatment, as it would send chronic, long term problems back to the primary care provider. This is similar to the current system where continued care is supposed to be done by the patient's "regular doctor". The emphasis is on primary care providing a long-term health relationship for you, the patients, so that those primary care providers will have a more in depth understanding of your particular needs. This new system will get those primary care offices closer to you as a patient and again secure a better understanding of you, the patient and hopefully, therefore, improve your health. Far too often, the patients go to "the ER", because they have not had the insurance to see a primary care, or there was too long a wait list to get in to see a primary care, or they couldn't get in because their schedule is too full, or the primary care is too far away, or the hours are inconvenient, or.... The list just seems to go on. The emphasis will be on getting more primary care offices where the people are, with transfer to more specialized care only as needed. This type of personal care relationship is especially lacking in rural and low-income areas. This new federal medicine system would particularly target those areas, so that care will be available where the patients are, not where bigger profits are to be made. A unique problem is that it is often difficult to start up a practice in a rural area, because that area may not have a large enough patient base to allow for a provider to succeed. A government system would ensure that care is available where it is needed, and since the provider is salary based, there will be no concern about seeing enough patients in order to prosper. Facilities would tend to grow and shrink based on the populations in those areas. A minimum health care presence would continue, based on both population and distances to care facilities, to ensure that rural areas are not left without care because those rural areas couldn't find a provider willing to live in their town. This would likely allow many smaller towns to keep more of their current population, as people wouldn't move away because of lack of health care. There would be a side benefit in that these facilities would inject more money, jobs and people into these rural communities. By having the facilities closer to the people, we again decrease reliance on Emergency Rooms. ER visits are a very expensive form of care and so it would decrease health care costs as the number of ER visits decreased. Increased reliance on primary care office visits would improve quality and decrease cost. If the offices are geographically convenient, accessibility would increase and problems would be treated when they are still minor, instead of waiting till they are very serious or even life threatening. If they are serious to begin with, then transport to a higher level of care will be done quickly and efficiently. Economically accessible and geographically accessible care will help improve health across the country.

Fed Med would also help to reduce redundancy in effort, facilities and personnel; with a desire to get the care to the people. But where exactly would the facilities be placed? A very quick way to get a federal system up and running would be to use current facilities, such as the VA, military facilities and Indian Health facilities. (Security concerns would need to be worked out before using some these facilities.) Extending hours to accommodate for the increased patient population would be a quick fix. Next step would be to purchase existing hospitals, particularly the ones that are struggling to remain open. Those purchases would be at current market rates. These purchases would only apply to facilities that wanted to sell, there would not be any eminent domain transactions. Many county and rural facilities would likely opt for this option as many are already having difficulties remaining open and this could reduce the strain on budgets for some local communities. There would still be a need to purchase some new facilities, these could be built on federal lands, possibly abandoned military facilities, where some infrastructure might already be available. The larger specialty facilities would not need to be built in the heart of large cities where land and infrastructure would be very expensive, but instead built some distance away where costs would be less and possibly equidistant between more than one major metropolitan area. These larger facilities would then have room for expansion, possibly to include research facilities. The key would be to keep as cost efficient as possible while providing care where it is needed.

Another major concern is that mental health care is woefully inadequate in the US now. There will need to be a large number of acquisitions of mental health facilities, because over the years more and more were shut down because of abuses in those facilities or lack of profit. There will be need for all types of mental health care facilities. There is need for out-patient clinics, short term care, dementia units, long term facilities, facilities for the homeless, substance abuse treatment centers and units for the criminally insane. The facilities will not just be warehouses to hold the mentally ill but will be treatment facilities with a goal of returning patients back to society. As mental health care improves, anticipate that less patients will be caught up in the criminal justice system. That a large number of "criminal types" are actually people with mental health problems and if these are recognized and treated we would likely have less criminals behind bars. Some of the current correctional facilities might be converted to treatment facilities, but with the goal of treating them to get back into society rather than just warehousing them, till they have completed their punishment. We will need to be creative in acquiring the many mental health facilities that we need.

One of the biggest specialty segments of our society that needs additional facilities is Obstetrics/gynecology and infant care. Lack of access to family planning results in too many unplanned pregnancies. Availability of OB/gyn clinics would allow more women to better control their reproductive life. This is especially true in our rural areas and inner cities. This results in the US have an unacceptably high rate of infant mortality for a developed country. Partly due to lack of specialty care in these areas, expectant mothers do not receive the pre-natal care that they need to assure healthy deliveries. This lack of pre-natal care often represents the missed opportunity to treat some maladies in the womb or the missed chance to plan for difficult deliveries. The long distances or drive times often decrease access for appropriate pre-natal care in rural areas. We need to have more obstetrics trained providers in the rural areas. We need to increase access to OB/gyn clinics for young women, who often will be lacking the insurance to obtain health care from commercial facilities. Hopefully by providing more access to prenatal care we would decrease infant mortality in the US. We must also tie infant care to these facilities to ensure that these children are all immunized and checked more closely to decrease our current rate of infant deaths. There is so much more we can and must do to improve the health and health statistics of our citizens. Federal medicine is the way that we could accomplish this goal. Placing care where the patients are, rather than just considering where the most profitable markets are, makes sense for the nation. A federal health care plan, such as I've discussed, could accomplish these goals.

Who Will Be Affected?

THE HEALTH CARE industry affects every person in the US, at some time in their life. Health care costs have made access to quality, affordable health care to become a thing of the past for too many people. Health insurance has now become a benefit of employment, a guaranteed benefit for those who are lower income or disabled, or a perk for those who can afford it. These groups represent the insured; those who have their insurance card, guaranteeing them access to health care. Unfortunately, for some of these people, even with that little card representing their insurance, this guarantee of health care often isn't the reality. Today, insurance often dictates who will provide your care, where you can receive your care, what care you will receive and how much you will be required to pay as well. Far too often, even insured patients are met with high costs of care, or they are often denied the care they need. Medicaid patients are often unable to receive specialty care, because there are no providers willing to accept their insurance; they are left with untreated illnesses often causing a continued decline in their health. Many with insurance have such high deductibles or co-pays that they don't seek medical care because it is still too expensive, even with insurance. Other patients may start off with insurance, but their illness or injury causes them to lose their insurance as they are no longer able to remain employed. For many of those unfortunate people, they often will not qualify for Medicaid because their income for the last 12 months was too high. Even worse is when someone has accumulated a home and retirement savings and then must spend it all on payment for their health care. (We are the only developed country that causes people to declare bankruptcy, to pay for health care. More than 40,000 people are forced to declare bankruptcy every year.) There is a huge number of people in the middle class who are stuck, they have high deductibles on top of paying high costs for their share of their insurance. Their first visits are paid out of pocket as they meet their deductible (until the deductible is met all costs are out of pocket.) One person I know had insurance payments of $13,200 per year for himself, his wife, and their one child. On top of this, his deductible is $12,000. He would have to pay $25,000 before his insurance even begins to cover his health care bills. The Affordable Care Act was established to get health insurance to more people with a promise that premiums would not increase appreciably. Unfortunately, the for-profit insurance companies now had a product that was a requirement for everyone and prices rose. Instead of just raising premiums 4-5% as was promised, some companies increased by 10, 20, 50, 100% (one report had plans going even higher.) The promise of less expensive was not the final result, as other commercial plans also increased their prices dramatically. A federal health plan would dispense with the need for health insurance, and the excessive costs associated with it. We need a new system that eliminates or reduces the need for health insurance. Administrative costs and profits in the insurance industry are some of the highest in the business world and recent profit numbers are some of the highest in several years for the insurance industry.

But why are other health care costs so high? In addition to the high costs of insurance, are the high costs of administration and management in a private or commercial hospital. The VA hospitals pay a top salary of about $400,000 per year to only a select number of specialty physicians. The average salary for CEOs in America's 4,000 hospitals is over $800,000. That is just the CEO's pay; then add all the other management personnel, the CFO, the CIO, the… and the list goes on. The top administrator pay is about $167,000 at the Veteran's Administration. Providing a federal medicine plan would cost far less on managerial staff salaries and therefore affect taxpayers and patients by reducing overall costs for health care.

A very important group that is affected by health care decisions are the providers themselves; the doctors, nurse practitioners, physician assistants, and nurses. This group, those people who provide direct care to the patients, is often left out of discussions regarding health care. A great example is that when the Affordable Care Act was passed, they failed to discuss the need for more providers to accommodate the new influx of patients, (this also happened at the VA, where there was a failure to increase providers as the Vietnam generation started to turn 60 and required more care and there were the soldiers returning from the middle east conflict.) An odd and yet fortunate timing was that the Affordable Care Act's start coincided with the great recession. There were many physicians who had planned to retire, but they stayed in practice because their savings were depleted by the recession. They stayed and continued to work and thus absorbed some of the bump of additional patients. (Sadly, the bump in patients was not as big as it might have been because even with insurance, deductibles and co-pays kept health care too expensive for many to enjoy.) The influx of additional patients was absorbed but the system is near capacity and the US still falls below recommended ratios of physicians to patients recommended by the World Health Organization. One plan currently being recommended is: "Medicare for all". If the plan were implemented, there would be an increase of 5-20% more patients, yet there is nothing in the plan to increase the number of providers. We need to consider the providers as a group that will be greatly affected by any health care discussions. We need to look at more than just costs as we evaluate possible solutions to our nation's health care problems. We will discuss some of the other aspects of a government supplied health care system in coming chapters.

To this point I have primarily discussed cost for patients, but let's look at other groups that are going to benefit from a federal health care system. Medicaid recipients continue to face several problems in our current system. There is a stigma attached to receiving safety net benefits, this stigma can influence a decline in care provided to a Medicaid patient. From groups that don't accept Medicaid insurance to subconscious bias in the provider; Medicaid patients are treated differently. Sometimes it's the knowledge that certain procedures or medicines won't be covered by the Medicaid insurance plan, so a provider just doesn't treat to the same standard as someone with good, commercial insurance. If there were one system with everyone receiving the same level of care, all care would be to the same level of excellence, not to the level of how the health care is paid for. All patients would receive the current standard of care that would be equal across the country. There would be no consideration of "what's covered on this plan?" No hesitation to give the best care to everyone, therefore the nation's health would improve.

An additional aspect of this federal medicine is that since it is an option available to everyone there would no longer be income caps to retain your coverage. Everyone would be covered! With income caps gone, people (especially single parents) would be able to return to work if they desired, they wouldn't lose health care benefits. A sense of forced poverty would be lifted. A person would no longer have to worry about maintaining Medicaid health care versus going to work and then having to pay for insurance to provide health care. There are many people who are working in the "gray economy", being paid under the table so that they can maintain benefits. This cheats the country from collecting taxes but also makes so that those individuals are not contributing to Medicare or social security for their future. We are inadvertently rewarding maladaptive behavior, those people working the gray economy can't move up the economic ladder for future benefits because they need to provide for an immediate need in the present. If a federal medical system were available we would dramatically improve this group's future.

This country lacks adequate mental health care! Those suffering from mental health issues are a group that would benefit dramatically. There are not enough facilities or providers in mental health care. We discussed the need for facilities in the last chapter. The huge need for additional providers is evident in too many of our current headlines. When we have another school shooting, where were the psychologists and trained counselors that might have identified the killer before the event occurred. We are concerned about substance abuse, but where are the treatment centers and psychiatrists and counselors to help them rid of their addiction. There is such a huge number of suicide deaths (particularly veterans), yet where are the counselors and psychiatric facilities to treat their depression. A federal medical system could focus on these groups and help to alleviate some of these problems. Mental health care has had a gradual decline since the fifties. Part of this was the outcry at how some patients were abused or mistreated in mental health facilities, often those facilities exhibiting bad behavior were closed leaving even less facilities to care for a growing population of mentally ill patients. Another aspect related to the decrease in the availability of mental health care is that it is just not as profitable as other specialties. Mental health care patients tend to require more intense and time-consuming treatment, but rarely require any expensive procedures. The result has been a steady decline in the number of mental health care facilities and an increase of untreated or undertreated individuals. There are estimates that there are at least 25% of the homeless having severe mental health issues that are not treated. Does the mental illness cause the homelessness or does homelessness cause mental health problems? It doesn't seem to matter, because if you are homeless you are not going to have an address to send your Medicaid card to, or a facility that is available during a time of psychological distress. Often, if they have a mental illness they may have trouble understanding how to get health insurance/Medicaid and then difficulty getting to any health care facilities. With a federal system, they automatically qualify and will be treated when they show up or if they are arrested. They will get their care as quickly as possible and may even be diverted from the criminal justice system. There are too many who are mentally ill that are sent to our prisons and jails. It is estimated that 64% of local jail inmates, 56% of state prisoners and 45% of federal felons are mentally ill. Having a federal medical system would likely reduce this incarceration rate. So with a federal medical we would reduce homelessness and crime. Mental health patients would be hugely improved with Fed Med. This would also include those suffering from substance abuse. 37% of alcoholics and 53% of drug addicts are reported to have additional (co-morbid) mental health issues. We are currently in an Opioid Crisis, yet we lack the treatment facilities to help people with addictions. Many of the treatment facilities that do exist; are far too expensive, lack effective treatment protocols or have excessive wait times to get into them. Fed Med would be able to address this problem, this lack of adequate mental health care facilities and providers.

A federal health care system would be able to channel resources to provide better mental health care to our population. By replacing a for-profit focus with emphasis only on the best health of our citizens, we can improve our country's health. Another sobering fact is the number of suicide deaths in our country. The current system does not do nearly enough to prevent suicide or treat depression. Because of this lack of care, it is estimated that 22 veterans die everyday due to suicide, and its not just veterans, we have roughly one physician who takes his own life daily as well. We worry about gun deaths and yet we fail to provide one of the strongest deterrents in the form of quality accessible mental health care. It is not just the mass shootings that would be prevented but also the huge numbers of suicides and crimes of passion. A federal health care system would help address and treat mental health care as our current system is not meeting this need.

Who else will be affected by a federal system? Only those who want to be in the system. There is a fear from some people that they would be required to use a federal system. Far from it, this system would allow more freedom. If you want to use the system, then do so. If you don't want to participate, there will be no requirement or penalty for non-participation. This would be the public system for health care, just as public schools are the public system for education.

However, there would be no compensation if you "opt out", you will always be able to access it whenever you want or need to. This would be the only government provided system, it would replace Medicaid and Medicare. Fed Med would provide a more affordable, more accessible health care system that has better outcomes and expanded services, especially mental health care. This Fed Med system would affect everyone who desired quality, affordable and accessible health care. It would be a health care system of the people... for the people.

Who Will Staff this New System?

OTHER HEALTH CARE plans do not address the question of who will staff a federal medical system. As I've discussed in the last chapter, the US does not have enough physicians, how would this system get the providers needed? There are several plans that want to add additional recipients of health care but there is nothing in these plans that discusses how to gain additional providers. We as a nation still do not meet WHO guidelines and recommendations for numbers or types of health care providers. We also have a problem, in that too many of our providers are over age 55, meaning that too many are within ten years of possible retirement, or are at increased risk of debilitating disease or death. Private industry is not able or has been unwilling to meet the need for more physicians. So, how could we increase the numbers of providers needed?

The federal government could simply increase the number of training positions available. This could be accomplished by either creating more federal teaching facilities or by requesting existing medical schools to increase the numbers of training spots for new Fed Med students. There are plenty of qualified applicants, yet we continue to limit the available number of spots to train doctors. This creates an artificial low supply and keeps demand high, therefore maintaining high salaries. It's time for the federal government to increase the number of providers instead of keeping the numbers low to justify high wages for the relatively low number of physicians. One thing that prevents many qualified applicants from pursuing a medical education is the high personal costs of training. The personal cost for many new physicians is often around $250,000 just for medical school, (it doesn't account for lost wages, undergraduate costs or interest.) This often forces new graduates to go to work for corporate medicine; the big hospitals, big medicine where they soon become just another employee, though one with special skills. These high costs are often prohibitive for many minority students, resulting in less diversity in our health care providers. Fed Med would equal the access for many more minorities and for lower income, qualified applicants. An increase in diversity would also help to decrease some of the mistrust toward health care found in some minority groups. Increasing diversity in and of itself is a laudable thing for our society to do; but improving the numbers of qualified providers is even more important. Paying for more providers would enhance our medical system by gaining a larger number of qualified applicants and ensuring that training was consistent with the needs of the nation. This could be rectified by having a system similar to the US Air Force manner of training pilots. If students were offered training with a follow-on requirement of service, would we be able to get more physicians to work in this new Fed Med? It works very well in the Air Force as pilots spend several years gaining experience that they may use to stay in the military for an entire career or to accumulate the experience needed to gain employment in commercial aviation. We need more physicians and a federal system could provide that additional supply that our nation demands.

In starting this new federal system there would necessarily be a transition period when there were current qualified physicians, residents and students who would be mixed with the new system trained providers. These "old system" individuals would need to be incentivized to participate in the new Fed Med system. This compensation could be in the form of paying off loans, cash payments or Career points (this will be explained later.) The desire to be a health care provider should not be penalized with exorbitant training costs. This system would need providers, and a federal health care system would need to make sure they were provided with the appropriate incentives to make the system work.

Training physicians currently requires a college degree, then medical school, then a residency training program where your specialty status is conferred and for some an additional fellowship, granting an even more specialized status. Much of medical training now occurs at Veterans Administration facilities; this training could now work under much closer relationship with civilian Federal facilities. A new option that might be considered is to grant a medical degree and then have physicians work as primary care providers and then go on to specialization after they have gained more experience in general medicine. If their time spent as general practice physicians was increased to possibly two or three years, they may find that they are more proficient at certain areas of interest in health care. Then after this increased experience in specialty care they would then get further training in that particular specialty, eventually being granted specialty status in the area that they are noted to be better at. If a provider desired training to be a specialist, one would get a choice in areas that the government needs, not in what was more lucrative to the individual. The choice of becoming specialized might also rest on accumulation of career points, a potential new concept for furthering an individual's career. These career points would reflect doing extra things to further your career. Some of those things might be: staying as a general primary care provider for a longer period of time, potentially it could reflect having served at a facility that is less than desirable to the average physician (a rural site, an inner-city location), willingness to serve as an emergency response team that would relocate to a crisis area such as hurricane response, acting as locum tenens to cover when a physician is ill, or incapacitated or on vacation. These are situations that are not always sought after by providers, they are the situations that would be rewarded with career points. These situations would better be covered by a Federal medicine program.

This novel manner of care would allow for increased experience in all physicians. Our country also has care providers that are not physicians. In a transitionary period, it should be allowed that Nurse practitioners and Physician assistants receive additional training and be granted the title of Doctor (MD) after completion of this training, with waiver of some training based on experience previously achieved. In the US training of providers on a continuous basis is currently done by the individual, Continuing Medical Education (CME) is accomplished at their cost and chosen by the doctor. Consideration of having weekly training done through federal facilities might improve the content of training for consistency, timeliness, and relevance to treatments. This training could also include instruction on new medications and procedures, as they are approved by the Food and Drug Administration, FDA. Maintenance and continuous updates in medical knowledge will thus be achieved.

Specialty training, as I have said, would be provided after gaining experience or particular specialty expertise is noted. Specialty training could be a reward for having worked in a rural area, overseas location, or other position that is difficult to fill. Specialty training would be provided based on the numbers and type of specialists needed by the federal medical system. People trained in a particular specialty may still be assigned to provide general care; if their specialty does not maintain a full schedule. Specialty training would be above and beyond recommendations for general physician requirements as recommended by the American Academy of Family Physicians (AAFP).

I've discussed physician health care providers, Individuals that would be like officers in the military and gain promotion commensurate with ability and time spent in this system. There would develop a pyramid of those who are the best in their specialty, leaders in their field and top managers as they best understand the care needs of patients. These "officers of medicine" will be deciding policy, establishing procedures, and evaluating the success of their therapeutic actions. They will be responsible for the direction of medical care in our country; rather than looking for profit, they will be looking at the optimal health of the people of this country.

These health providers will also require the assistance of nursing staff and technicians. These personnel could be supplied with a rank structure similar to that of warrant officers in the military, or in a separate promotion pool. There should also be an education path to allow for change to provider track if desired by the individual. If desired, a blending of these career paths might be appropriate. But the use of a merit and timed progression in rank will be used for this group as well.

A third group is all the other ancillary staff. These would be the administrative staff, clerks, maintenance, cooks, housekeeping, etc. This group could be likened to enlisted people in the military. These people generally are not as highly trained, but still provide much of the work done in a health care facility. This group could be filled by our Nation's young people. Allowing the group that is most affected by unemployment to have access to a huge labor pool. A provision could be added that, by performing this work for four years, participants would be rewarded with tuition and books to public universities, colleges, and trade schools. This action would help not just the individual, but also society, by providing a new generation of college educated community members. They would continue to push our knowledge base forward and maintain the US as a world leader in technology.

We would have a new renaissance in technological prowess. This service to our country will also engender greater pride in their country. This opportunity to serve your country outside of military service could also be used as a path to citizenship. The expectation would be that this service opportunity would not be a career; but that it would likely be used as a stepping stone to education.

I've described this government health care system as being similar to that of the military and the public health service. A hierarchy of doctor "officers", with the majority of the personnel being at a level similar to that of enlisted personnel in the US military. For certain technical jobs, there could also be a level of personnel similar to warrant officers in the US military. They would have specialized knowledge, but not the prolonged training of the doctors.

The pay and benefits would be similar to a hybrid of current military and government service pay systems. One new aspect that I would add would be Career Points. Not every location will be considered ideal, or certain specialties might be perceived as less desirable. The individuals who are assigned to these duties or locations would be provided with extra incentives that I would call "career points". These points might be accumulated and then redeemed to get a guaranteed, location, specialty, or even an increase in retirement pay. Or they may receive extra consideration for promotion. An example might be an individual serving in psychiatry (currently one of the lowest paid specialties) receiving one career point per year. After accumulating five career points, the provider might decide to utilize them to change her specialty or get a move to her preferred location. A person working in a large, popular city might receive no career points and be subject to placement in a different city or specialty, based on the needs of the government. Another aspect of my planned Fed Med is that after a person has completed the minimum payback time, they could leave Federal service and work in the private sector or change career fields entirely.

The numbers of providers and staff members would be based on government needs. Numbers and types of specialties would be based on needs at that time. A provider might start in one specialty but move to another medical specialty based upon needs of the government in a certain area. As a member gains more experience, they may be channeled into management, academics, research, or policy. As the system evolves, changes would be made to ensure that we are maintaining optimal health for our patients.

A crucial aspect of this system is that it would be more responsive to crisis, loss, or emergency than anything our country currently has in place. If an emergency arises, such as a hurricane or other natural disaster, we could quickly take necessary personnel from an unaffected area and assign them temporarily to this crisis location with high needs. In a war, we could quickly backfill stateside base locations, allowing those military personnel needed for wartime duties to go to wartime locations. In addition, with a loss of a key provider in any location, this system would have the ability to quickly find a long-term replacement. This system could also better allow for vacations, training, sabbaticals, illnesses, or other types of loss of personnel. These vacancies could be filled quickly and effectively by experienced personnel in short-term situations. Again, by making oneself available for these rapid need relocations, these staff could generate career points. The providers and staff would be able to make many choices but, ultimately, assignments will be based on need and the current requirements of the government's Fed Med system. This system would be able to evolve and change relative to its utilization by the people in this country and the changes that occur in medical therapy. Fed Med would be the best way to ensure a well trained medical community that is responsive to the needs of the Nation. With its emphasis on primary care providers, access to care will be enhanced and the overall health of the Nation will be improved.

Who Would NOT Benefit?

ONLY TWO GROUPS would likely not benefit from this system: large commercial medical systems and health insurance companies. While they would not be shut down if our country were to adopt Fed Med, those for-profit companies would likely become much smaller. The insurance companies and large medical systems would be necessary during any transition to this new government health care system, and they would continue for anyone choosing to continue with a private system.

Fed Med is not intended to replace them. However, federal payment for health care would be shifted to federal facilities and providers. For-profit hospitals and insurance will remain for those who choose to stay with private health care. However, similar to our public education system, most people would find the public option, Fed Med, to be a cost-effective option providing quality care.

These two groups are likely to resist adoption of a government health care system. Health care is a big business and there would be claims of how bad government systems are in the world, despite the evidence to the contrary. There would be all sorts of tactics used to prevent consideration of government facilities. They would likely try scare tactics to suggest that there would be "death panels" and inferior care and long wait times and worse outcomes. Yet evidence from countries that have government supplied care are overwhelmingly supportive of the US switching to government provided care. Problems in other countries usually result when the government underfunds these systems, then blame the system for not being able to provide quality care. (Just as public education is blamed for bad scores by students when the schools are woefully underfunded.) A likely outcome of discussing a possible change in the medical care system is that there will be a large surge in lobbyist activity and campaign contributions. Calm rational analysis of the ideas and facts presented in this book could help to dispel some of those arguments. There is far too much money in the current medical system and the large corporations will be reluctant to give that up. Anticipate the statements and questions, research the concepts presented and recognize that the benefits will be for the people of this nation not for the corporations.

What are some other benefits of Fed Med?

A NATIONAL HEALTH system, Fed Med, would provide multiple solutions, not simply improved access and reduced cost. Fed Med, by not being tied to a requirement of generating a profit, would be able to provide better care at a more affordable cost. The mission statement would be: To provide care resulting in the best health of the people living in the US. This is often in opposition to what seems to commonly be a mission statement in the business world: To provide the best care possible at the lowest cost. The difference in focus is the emphasis on health as opposed to cost. The greatest profit will occur when the goods and services paid for by the health care corporation are at the lowest cost. As a CEO of an insurance company recently told me, "Remember, we are a for-profit company."

A public option of universal health care, Fed Med, will look first and foremost, to provide the highest quality health care, as opposed to focusing on profit being the motivator of providing care. The benefit of a government health care program is that we can achieve quality health care while reducing costs, because the profit motive will be removed. Cost will decrease because there is no drive for increased numbers of visits, because the goal is improved health. Cost will also decrease because the push to perform expensive procedures, without clear need, will diminish. With a guaranteed salary, as opposed to being paid in volume (per patient), physicians will no longer be motivated to pursue higher cost options, they will be motivated to act as an advocate for optimal health of their patients. The sole intent is to achieve the best health outcome for all of their patients without regard to generating more profit.

Cost will continue to decrease as there is a stronger push towards preventive care, decreasing some of today's top killers: heart disease, type II diabetes, and cancer. Renewed and better funded focus on mental health care, including well trained and ample numbers of providers in mental health care will also decrease overall health care costs. A strong focus on mental health care will help better address some other top concerns, such as homelessness, substance abuse, gun violence, and abnormal behaviors that result in incarceration in our jails and prisons.

A large cost reduction will come from a decrease of redundant lab work and imaging procedures because reports from differing facilities and providers, as well as excessive tests being done primarily to protect the provider from a fear of malpractice will all be available in one place. With one charting system; tests, labs, and imaging results will be readily available to any physician or facility in any location. This will negate the need to rerun a test or scan that may have just been completed days or even hours earlier.

If we implement a federal fund pool to reimburse patients negatively impacted by their health care, individual malpractice insurance would no longer be necessary. Individuals who are affected would instead receive funds from this pool as recommended by arbitration.

As you can see, cost reduction will be accomplished by a Federal Medical system. And, as they often say in television ads, "But wait - - there's more!" We have seen how access will be spread to locations where care is needed, as opposed to primarily being located where the highest profit can be made. The focus is on where the patients are and providing them with quality health care. We have seen how there will be more providers, with an emphasis on primary and preventive care. We have seen how there will be an increased emphasis on mental health, a critical and often missed area of a person's overall health. What other benefits could we anticipate with a Federal Medical system?

A single Electronic Health Record (EHR) system would provide numerous benefits. As mentioned just moments ago, a patient's records would now be accessible from anywhere in the country. If a person moves or is travelling, their records would still be available to any provider they choose to see within the Fed Med system. This was one of the original intents when paper charting progressed to electronic records. However, this intended benefit has been lost in the implementation of this system because the different record systems don't communicate well with one another.

With a universal EHR system, past medical problems, previous surgeries, and all known allergies to medicines would be instantly accessible by other providers, without having to take the extensive time to redo a new history every time a patient sees a new doctor or specialist. This also greatly decreases the risk of missing a forgotten item. The more complex a patient's health becomes, the more difficult it is to remember who they've already provided with the information. Critical details would no longer potentially be undocumented. This universal system would ensure access to previous labs and diagnostic results. This would reduce unnecessary repetition of tests and there would be immediate comparisons to previous results so a physician could see trends, or significant changes or differences, in results. If a problem was found with a particular medication, the treatment could quickly be stopped on all patients, decreasing further potential concerns caused by the offending medication. The prevalent opiate crisis has shown how some patients travel from one physician to another, without the ability to be detected because most reporting doesn't cross state lines. This universal system would provide all physicians with instant access to track any controlled medication, greatly decreasing any opportunity for patients to doctor shop. In addition to detecting these potential offenders, this records system could greatly help physicians monitor appropriate opiate use by a patient. The potential for early detection of escalating use, and potential abuse of opiates, greatly increases, allowing physicians to more quickly refer their patient to mental health to get the appropriate treatment. Another clear and extremely relevant example of how we can utilize this entire program to drastically improve patient care.

In addition to being used to track a patient's personal health records and results, this EHR system could also have a private mode. This mode would only allow certain identifying information to exist if a patient so desired. Patients would then be able to securely carry their critical medical information with them for physicians and emergency medical professionals to access if needed. This record system could be similar to a credit card with a chip reader. The patient would have their information, but it wouldn't be fully accessible by the federal system without additional approvals from the patient, or only critical information would be immediately available. By utilizing a private mode in patients' records, aggregate information, without each patient's personal information being included, would allow research to determine which treatments are most effective for a specific patient demographic. This research capability would allow for retrospective pharmaceutical and treatment studies to be accomplished in days and weeks, instead of months and years. This could help shape care decisions to the most appropriate care instead of simply the most profitable care. With this incredibly powerful tool, we could better determine what care, treatment, and medications are truly the most effective and beneficial to improving patient health. It would remove the barrier of physicians having to select only generic medications or the least expensive treatment because cost would no longer be the driving factor in their decision-making process, your optimal health is the goal that counts. In addition, further research could be done to see if there was an alternative method or treatment that is even more cost effective. The nearly instant access to larger demographic groups could greatly increase the statistical certainty that we are providing the best care for our patients.

In discussing research, a federal system would also have greater influence on the direction of research. Nutritional supplements often have no scientific research to back up their claims, or at best, flawed studies taken from small populations. The FDA was created, in part, to deal with questionable treatments. With a Federal Medical system, the studies could easily be done. This would prove whether some of these products are truly beneficial, of no effect, or potentially dangerous. One particular group of studies that has not been done, yet is desperately needed, is the study of the effectiveness of marijuana, THC, and CBDs. Initial studies could begin with simply a history of use and move on to determine if there may be a correlation between past marijuana use and improved health, or negative effects on that patient's health. Studies could then be designed with controls to determine marijuana's potential value as a medical treatment, helping to determine effective doses and the best means of administering the substance. Research would shift to a basis of factual, proven outcomes without any bias towards gaining profit. With this research being more strictly based on health outcomes, as opposed to profitability, many more health care treatments and medicines could be evaluated. The emphasis would shift to the whole person, not just the research goals.

There are several other benefits that are often not

mentioned when discussing universal health care, such as Fed Med. The benefits to business, employees, and the economy could be tremendous. Currently, many corporations spend huge sums of money for their employees' health insurance benefits. On average, this benefit is costing the business $12,000 per employee, per year. If employers no longer had to cover the cost of health insurance for their employees, the savings could then go to higher wages for their employees, investment in or expansion of their business, or, for corporations, being able to pay out more in their stock dividends. There are also many small businesses that can't afford, or are not required to carry, insurance for their employees. As a result, many qualified workers can't or won't work in a small business. Suddenly, small businesses would be able to be more competitive regarding benefits for employees.

From an employee's perspective, Fed Med would be a very welcome benefit for them. Not only would they no longer have to pay into their own health insurance, but they could now expect to see pay increases from their employers who now have more money available in their benefits pools. Many employees would be afforded the opportunity to request increased pay. If they were denied their desired increase, they would now have the freedom to change jobs without the concern of losing their employer provided insurance benefits. Many employees could potentially decide to start their own businesses, or work shorter hours, without needing to be concerned about having or losing coverage for health care. In addition, the American employee's benefits package would be less costly, thus making employees more competitive with employees in the rest of the developed nations.

The potential positive impact on our nation's economy is enormous. By getting rid of the cost of insurance, $1 trillion will be pumped back into the US economy, as businesses and individuals would no longer have to pay for their insurance premiums. Spending on housing, vehicles, and personal goods would spur the economy. Goods and services would likely cost less, and exports should, in theory, increase, as the cost to make products in the US is decreased by lower labor costs. Eliminating the cost of insurance will decrease an employee's benefit package cost and therefore labor costs to produce goods or services is decreased and this should increase sales domestically and around the world.

By shifting from a primarily for-profit system, to a system that guarantees quality care, individuals no longer need worry about if or how their care will be provided. We will no longer delay seeking medical care because we can't afford it. Therefore, we will be much more likely to get care before a minor complaint turns into a life or death situation.

The benefit of changing to a government supplied system also includes the great benefit of equalizing everyone in our country. This benefit would be available to every person, regardless of age, gender, or income. It would be available to every person, whether or not they are employed. This system would also build community involvement and patriotism by having more people serving their nation through the medical service, in addition to our current military service. A Federal Medical system, by definition, is of the people – for the people – by the people. This system would not be mandatory, but it would provide every person living in our country with a viable option to quality health care. This enhances every person's freedom of choice and opportunity, which is supposed to be inherent in our great nation.

What You Can Do

YOU ARE YOUR best patient advocate. As such, you need to be proactive in your health care. Take responsibility to help make yourself as healthy as possible. Most of the time, this means following the preventive medicine recommendations provided to you. It isn't always necessary to access a medical provider to maintain good health; but when you need to get care from a trained provider, you should be able to get that care.

Some basics for physical well-being are well known, and well worth repeating. Eat a healthy diet; follow the recommendations of the FDA, CDC, and the Agriculture Department. This is where you should start; balancing intake of protein, fats, and carbohydrates. Usually this will include recommendations for fruits and vegetables, meats and dairy, and breads and other starches. Try to limit your sugar intake, as this usually equates to too many calories. Special diets with religious or personal influences may restrict certain nutrients; find out about alternatives and use them as appropriate. Evaluate calorie content based on your needs, and again, avoid excess sugars and fats as they are very calorie dense: many calories in a small amount of food. Beware of the many special diets for weight loss, as they are often gimmicks. They restrict calories by excluding one type of macro-nutrient which is usually not replaced by a compensating food that is allowed in the new diet. Weight gain and loss tend to be a simple balance of calories ingested (eating) versus calories out (exercise and activity). Often a moderate decrease in portions and walking thirty minutes every day is enough to lead to a healthier you. Exercise is one of the keys to good health, it should include aerobic, strengthening and balance training. Don't forget to remain hydrated! Make water your primary fluid choice, too many people are getting too many empty calories through their drink choices. One beverage to be especially careful of is alcohol. Recommendations are to limit consumption to 4-10 "standard drinks" per week, with no more than two drinks on any one day. Excessive use of alcohol is one form of substance abuse, it can be a detriment to both physical and mental health. Tobacco is one of the greatest detriments to good health. This one behavior tends to be most responsible for decreasing your longevity, and to decreasing your quality of life. If you want to be a good patient advocate for yourself…DON'T SMOKE. If you need help to stop smoking, contact your doctor.

Some things you can do for your mental health are to avoid narcotics and illicit drugs. Sounds reminiscent of the "just say NO!" campaign, but it really is true. Over 60,000 people died of narcotic causes in the last year on record. Other thoughts on mental health care would be my recommended coping mechanisms to help prevent depression and anxiety. These aren't meant to treat more severe cases of depression or anxiety but can be helpful as a guide to thinking more clearly and maintaining a positive mood.

1. HAVE FUN! Take time to enjoy life and take a break from all the worries. You need some "me time" daily to help from being overwhelmed by the day to day pressures. Life is supposed to be lived, don't just exist by living out a "life sentence"

2. EXERCISE The stressors of daily life will build up the fight or flight response in your body, let that pent-up energy out. Go for a walk, the movement will start as an energy release and then change to a relaxing rhythmic movement that will calm your mood.

3. TALK TO SOMEONE Allow yourself to verbally vent, get it off your chest, share your concerns with

someone else. This action will help you to know that others care about you and give you some possible solutions to your problem.

4. GOALS If you have a focus to your life, most people feel they are more in control of their life. Decide what you want to have, or what you want to do in your life. Look at what gives your life a sense of purpose. Once you've decided on your goals, come up with a plan to accomplish your goals. Society has some goals for everyone; Get a job, get married, buy a house, and raise a family. That set doesn't work for everyone, so look at what you want out of life and go after that goal. Don't sell yourself short, try for the goal. If you fail, then look for a possible alternative. But first decide what is truly important to you, then go for that goal.

As you can see, you are your most important patient advocate. There is much more you can do for your own health care. Often, we engage in activities that are not in our best interest. When engage in recreational activities, ensure that appropriate safety equipment is used. Recognize that some activities are inherently dangerous and weigh the risks and benefits before engaging in that activity. In addition, evaluate safe practice in sexual activity, no matter what your orientation, engage in activities in as safe a manner as possible. Many of the illnesses affecting us result from our behaviors and choices. The government continually studies what is causing problems in our health, it is our responsibility to learn and follow these recommendations to ensure we attain the best health possible. Research how to improve your life and act on the recommendations.

You can also do more. Work to get better medical healthcare for everyone! During election cycles, look at the candidates that will help to improve health care. Do your research and vote. Contact your elected representatives and let them know how important health care is to you. Write letters to the editor, discussing issues in health care you feel strongly about. Go to meetings and discuss your concerns. Join organizations that will help you to achieve your health care goals. Join a political party and make them understand your position on health care. (Being a member of a political party is often the only way you get to express yourself in primary elections.) Be involved, be the best patient advocate for your own health and vote to get the health care system that you deserve! We deserve to have the best health possible, it is time for us to push our government to perform their responsibility and improve the health of every American.